THE
BIG 5 OF
YOUTH
WELLNESS

EVERYTHING YOUR DOCTOR
WANTS YOU TO KNOW

DR. SHEUN ADE-ALADE

TABLE OF CONTENTS

PART ONE
SEXUAL HEALTH

PART TWO
RELATIONSHIPS

PART THREE
MENTAL HEALTH

PART FOUR
A HEALTHY LIFESTYLE

PART FIVE
COMMON MEDICAL CONDITIONS

ACKNOWLEDGEMENTS

Many thanks to God Almighty who gave me the grace to put this book together during one of the busiest periods in my life. He remained my stronghold in those times when I felt confused as a young adult who could not tell her left from her right.

Special thanks goes to my wonderful husband, Prince Olukunle Ade-Alade who remains my pillar of support.

I express my love to my boys –Treasure, Gaius, Isaac and Moses. They are my strongest motivation for writing this book.

I'll like to thank my parents, Dr. and Mrs. Fasanmade who imbibed in me qualities that turned me into a healthy adult.

I'll like to appreciate Dr. Shola Ezeokoli who has mentored me through this process. You are a wonderful coach and it has been lovely to work with you.

DISCLAIMER

This book is written to inform the reader about common issues facing young people. It is not to be used as a medical reference to diagnose, treat or prevent any mental and medical health conditions.

The information in this book does not represent best medical practice or the guidelines for treatment of medical and mental health conditions.

The author or the publisher holds no responsibilities for the improper use of this book or any consequences arising from such use.

The author disclaims liability for any direct or indirect, incidental or consequential damages or losses that may result either directly or indirectly from the use of this book.

INTRODUCTION

There are so many issues facing young people today.

The transition period from childhood to young adulthood involves an interplay of hormones and emotions. Trying to balance these interplays with life challenges as young people take up more responsibilities can be quite difficult.

Within a 12-month period, mental health disorders among people in the twenties was 19.8% (men) and 32.4% (women).

On the average, a young person has been in contact with a professional for problem directly or indirectly relating to their mental health.

Issues causing low mood and anxiety in young people are quite different from those causing the same in adults.

If these issues are identified and tackled from a preventive point of view, this would go a long way in curbing the rising tide of mental health issues facing young adults in our world today.

This book is written differently, combining social, mental and medical issues in one place. It also provides journaling prompts after each section. Journaling can help readers take responsibility for their well-being and also help with self-reflection to find out how they can help themselves overcome some of these issues.

With concise and easy to read chapters, this book is not only for young people but for those who love them and seek to understand them better; Parents, teachers, and anyone who works with young people.

TIPS FOR PARENTS

As a family doctor, I have had the opportunity of speaking to parents of young persons during consultations.

Young people can be difficult to deal with especially as they go through their teenage years. They are sometimes confused at this stage, unsure whether to act like adults or children.

They would like to attain independence but at the same time need the support of loved ones. This period can also have an impact on their parents.

Young people want to feel listened to, they want parents to share in their happiness and also to be there when they are down.

This book will also help parents understand their young adults better: not only in the aspect of their mental health but also regarding medical conditions common to young adults.

It is also important to note that this period can also be challenging for parents of young adults, so maintaining a healthy lifestyle and taking adequate care of yourself as a parent will be helpful for everyone.

PART ONE
SEXUAL HEALTH

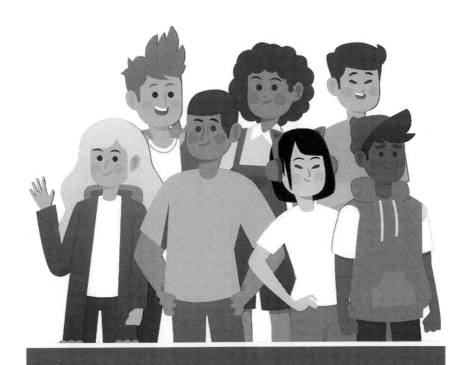

1

UNPROTECTED SEX

When youths say they have had unprotected sex they think this is just because they have not used condoms. We all know that condoms offer protection from falling pregnant or having infections transmitted through sex. Unprotected sex, however, goes beyond not using condoms or other forms of protection. It reaches to intangible things that have been left unprotected, issues that are beyond the physical.

A lot of questions remain unanswered when unprotected sex happens. Questions such as:

- Has your conscience been protected or your wishes been protected? Maybe you secretly wished you had waited until a certain age to have sex but you find yourself being lured.
- Do you lose your self-esteem and body image after having sex? There is a thin line between love and hate. When you are not fully ready for sex physically or emotionally, guilt and low self -esteem can set in easily thereafter.

A good number of young people have an idea about when they want to start having sex but what happens when you are unexpectedly placed in a vulnerable position? Vulnerable situations are almost always not planned for.

What do you do when placed in a vulnerable spot?

You have to be able to identify what vulnerable spots are. A raging night party? In a secluded room with your boyfriend? When under the influence of alcohol? At that point you have to deal with this by realising you are in a vulnerable state and think about what to do as soon as possible.

A lady once paid a visit to her boyfriend in the university hostel. The boyfriend then started to make attempts to have sex with her. They were alone in the room. She did not want to but she thought it would be shameful if she shouted out for help in a boys' hostel. She didn't want to make a scene.

What happened? She reluctantly gave in. That was a form of rape but the situation she found herself in, left her vulnerable. This eventually led to a breakup of that relationship.

Sometimes as a young person, thinking through possible vulnerable situations can help you know what to do if you were to find yourself in one. You may also be able to think about exit routes out of such situations without being raped.

Even though you love your boyfriend/girlfriend, there are consequences of unprotected sex like an unplanned pregnancy or a sexually transmitted infection. In addition, anxiety and stress can follow concerns about the above.

More young people are waiting to have sex and that is the best approach. This may sound outdated but it is the ideal. It has been shown that people who engage in sex soon after their first date or within the first month have the worst relationship outcome.

If you have had unplanned and unprotected sex, contact your nearest sexual health clinic or see your family doctor.

Recognize that having a missed period is usually the first sign of getting pregnant. It is therefore important to get help as soon as possible. If you have had unprotected sex, don't keep it to yourself. Please seek help. Not speaking to anyone about your concerns can put you in a more vulnerable position.

PREVENTING UNPROTECTED SEX

Remember, you have the right to say no to having sex at any time, irrespective of who is involved.

Protected sex is safe sex. Protection starts with knowing whether you are in the right relationship at the right time.

It starts with spotting potential vulnerability before the situation arises and knowing how to take action should you find yourself in such situation. Protection is protecting what really matters to you.

Avoiding risk may not be totally possible but here are some tips for reducing risk of unprotected sex:

1. Keep your phone charged at all times.
2. Set boundaries early enough on your date. Set clear communication about your reasons for not wanting to go into sex at this stage.
3. Try to set aside your emotions to act physically against being lured into sex.

2

GENITAL WARTS

A lot of young people worry about having had some genital warts at one time or the other. Genital warts are mostly found in women between the ages of 20 to 24 years and in men between the ages of 25 to 34 years. They are crops of growth caused by infection with the Human Papillomavirus (HPV).

Although there are many types of HPV viruses, the HPV-types 6 and 11 cause over 90% of genital warts. They are commonly sexually transmitted and can usually be found in the genital area i.e. around the penis and/or vagina.

They can also be found around the back passage, the mouth, and the neck of the uterus. They usually have a cauliflower-like appearance but may also appear flat or thick and horn-like. They can show up as a crop of growths or as a single growth.

The infection might not begin to show symptoms until after about three months. However the incubation period can range from three weeks to eight months.

It is important to recognise that if you have the genital form you might not show any external or physical symptoms.

It can be frightening for young people to notice a growth in the genital area. If you think you have genital warts, the first thing to note is that this is not cancer, nor does it mean you will develop cancer.

One third of cases do not need treatment as they disappear on their own within six months.

There are treatments available for genital warts. Based on the location of the warts, freezing treatments may be preferable. Freezing treatment is using liquid nitrogen to freeze and remove the warts.

There are also creams and solutions available by prescription.

Examples of creams include Podophyllotoxin and Imiquimod 5% cream.

Since genital warts are transmitted through sex, if you have genital warts, your partner should be seen for a check-up.

It is important to note that condom use can prevent HPV in up to 70% of cases. This is because HPV can infect other areas that are not covered by condoms e.g. other areas of genital skin.

3

CONTRACEPTION

This is a very important topic because if you're not planning to get pregnant and it happens, you can and will experience a series of life-changing events.

I used to know a lady when I was growing up. She always wanted to be a lawyer. She began the coursework required to attain a law degree. But mid-way, she got pregnant unexpectedly. The supposed father of the baby did not want to take any responsibility. This drained her physically and emotionally and being in a developing country, she did not have any support systems to rely on. Now having to care for a child as a single mum, she was forced to quit her immediate dreams of becoming a lawyer.

A planned pregnancy causes changes to your body, your feelings and your family; an unexpected pregnancy can bring about even more changes.

Becoming pregnant unexpectedly can be devastating and bring on a lot of negative consequences, depending on one's individual situation.

Apart from the pregnant person herself, parents or caregivers can feel shame or disappointment as the result of an unwanted pregnancy. The fear of a young person getting pregnant can bring a lot of anxiety to parents of sexually active young people.

Some young people think that having one episode of sex cannot lead to pregnancy but that is not the case.

Staying away from having sex is the safest method of contraception. This can keep you from having unwanted surprises and sexually transmitted infections.

Remember, You have the right to say 'No!'

There are different types of contraception available :

1. Condoms: A rubber sheath used over the penis to prevent exchange of body fluids during intercourse. They are easy to use but it is important that they are used appropriately.

Condoms do not protect against all forms of sexually transmitted infections (or STI) such as herpes and genital warts which can be spread through skin to skin contact.

2. The pill: These are artificial versions of the female hormones oestrogen and progesterone (naturally produced by the ovaries). There are 2 main types of pills; the oestrogen only and the combined pill. The combined pill contains both oestrogen and progesterone. They work mainly by blocking the natural forms produced by the ovaries. Note that they do not protect against STDS.

3. IUD: An IUD (or intrauterine device) is a small T-shaped device that is placed in the womb. The good thing about this is that it can last for several years. Depending on the type of device, they offer protection over a range of three years to ten years. They are small in size, and cannot be felt.

4. Implant: The implant is a small plastic rod containing artificial hormones that is placed under the skin of your upper arm. This can protect you from pregnancies for up to three years. The good thing is that you do not need to have to remember to take pills every day with the implant.

5. The injection: The shot or injection is a type of hormone called medroxyprogesterone (commonly called Depo-Provera). This usually lasts for 2 to 3 months. It may cause lighter periods and some young people may experience weight gain.

6. The patch: The patch is also a hormone in the form of ethinyl estradiol/norelgestromin. The patches can be applied to dry skin on the lower stomach below the waistline, the upper buttocks or the hips. They generally combine two hormones called oestrogen and Progestin. The hormones work with the ones which are produced naturally by your body.

It is worn for three weeks and then removed for a week. During the week off, you should get your period. You have to remember to apply and remove it on time. These are not as reliable as the IUD and the implant due to user error; forgetting to apply it or applying it wrong. They may even fall off without the user's knowledge.

The different methods can be discussed with your health care provider who will help you choose which is best for you, as they all have their pros and cons.

4

HPV AND THE HPV VACCINE

You most likely would have heard about or received the HPV vaccine. HPV stands for human papillomavirus (See earlier topic about genital warts). People get HPV infections primarily by having sex with someone who has the virus. HPV infection is one of the most common infections spread through having sex. It is a cause of cervical cancer.

The HPV vaccine is made by artificially producing viruses that share the same features as the human version. When you receive the vaccine, your body produces what we call antibodies. Antibodies then act as a guard against possible future exposure to the virus.

In the UK, the HPV vaccine is given to all young people in year 8 (usually aged 12-13 years). It can also be given in young adults and older adults up to 45 years old.

Some young people worry about side effects of the vaccine. Minor side effects from vaccines are common and they generally last a few days at most. You may experience mild reactions such as pain or redness in the arm where you have been injected. You may also experience a headache, a low-grade fever, tiredness, nausea or muscle pains. These symptoms do not last long.

Some people think that only girls need the vaccine. However, boys also need the vaccine as they can get warts and infections which can easily be passed from one person to another.

There are many forms of the HPV but the good thing is that the vaccine helps protect against ones that cause most HPV cancers.

It is important to note a lot of careful studies have been done to make sure the vaccine is safe. And contrary to popular belief, the HPV vaccine does not increase your tendency to have sex.

5

RAPE

Rape is a type of sexual assault usually involving sexual intercourse or other form of sexual penetration carried out against a person without their consent. It involves penetration of another person's vagina, anus, or mouth with a penis or other object.

Studies show that young people are about four times more likely to be victims of rape in any form than women in all other categories.

Men can also be raped by women or other men. Many cases of "loss of virginity" such as by a 12 year old boy to an 18 year old woman are actually rape cases. This chapter will focus on the more common form of rape, which is that inflicted on a female by a male. It is important to know that anyone forcing you to have any form of sex without your consent is counted as rape.

DATE RAPE

Date rape is a common form of rape. In this case, the victim is usually a friend or an acquaintance of the perpetrator. In some cases of date rapes, you may be in a romantic relationship but the difference is that you do not agree to having sex with your date. A lot of fear and shame may follow young people after a date rape as they probably knew their attacker.

Take this scenario: A 19 year old girl is invited to a party by some friends. It is a house party, and she is dancing and having a good time. At some point, a drink is shoved into her hand and she unsuspectingly takes a swig, not realising that the drink has been "spiked" with one of the many "date rape drugs" available illegally. Everything is fuzzy and the next thing she knows is that she is waking up with blood on her clothes.

Or another scenario:

Two people go out on a date. They have a good time. The man asks for sexual intercourse. The woman refuses. He forces himself on her.

These are both date rape scenarios and are unfortunately not uncommon. Many people have the impression that being raped is being dragged into a dark alley by a smelly stranger or group of strangers. This can lead to confusion in date rape cases when it comes to reporting. The lady may feel as though she "brought it on herself". This is NEVER the case as rape is ALWAYS the fault of the rapist.

Rape is not being "dragged into the bush". Rape is not always by strangers in the dark. It can perpetrated by people that we know. Date rape can be largely influenced by alcohol or illicit drugs. Alcohol can lower inhibition in both partners leading to poor decision making, as well as bodily changes that can disable a person from fighting off an attacker.

Here are some tips to reduce the risk of rape:

1. It is better to attend a party with friends than go alone. You might also want to stay with the group.

2. Stay aware of your surrounding at all times and avoid being somewhere alone with your date.
3. Never leave your drink unattended. If you need to attend the ladies, get a new drink in a new glass when you get back.

If you have been raped:

1. Do not take a shower even though that might be the only thing that you want to do.
2. Speak to a responsible older adult in your life immediately.
3. Go to the hospital and involve the police early.
4. Seek help from a therapist in order to work through the trauma.
5. Trust your feelings and don't minimise what you have gone through.
6. Call (a helpline) for assistance.

JOURNALING ON SEXUAL HEALTH

1. What are my concerns when it comes to sexual health?

2. How comfortable am I with talking about issues relating to sexual health with my parents, carers and loved ones?

3. What further information do I need?

4. When there are issues relating to sexual health, where are five places I could get the right advice and help?

PART TWO
RELATIONSHIPS

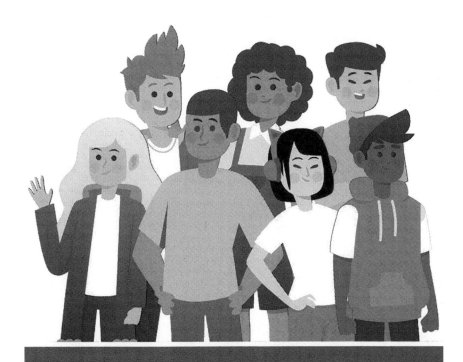

1

INTERPERSONAL VIOLENCE

Interpersonal violence is a form of violence between persons. This can happen within family or individual relationships or even in a larger community.

Interpersonal violence can result from behaviour exhibited by a person in order to exercise power and control over another person or persons. The result is that one can feel fearful and intimidated.

Emotional abuse is a form of interpersonal violence. It is defined as behaviour that causes psychological trauma or stress.

This can take the form of control and manipulation that can seem intangible. An example of this can be someone telling you that you are not good enough, you cannot be friends with them, or that you do not meet up to a certain standard.

Emotional abuses may not accompany other kinds of abuse but in many cases can follow physical or even sexual abuse.

Of note, physical and sexual abuse, being more obvious, are much easier to identify,

How can you identify emotional abuse/violence?

- Controlling behaviour, making demands and expecting them to be fulfilled.
- Requiring immediate responses from calls or texts.
- Giving excessive gifts with the implication that the individual may lose if they left the relationship or friendship.
- Trying to make you feel shame for your mistakes.
- Pulling you down when you feel like making your opinions known.
- Name calling, abusive jokes or insulting your looks.

What do I need to do when faced with violence of any form?

Once you recognise that you are facing one form of violence or another, the next step is to decide your response. A lot of young people respond to violence in a way that can most likely trigger further violence.

Among young people, provocation is a common starting point for eventual violence. Someone does something offensive to you and the next thing you want to do is fight back.

The first step in dealing with interpersonal violence is winning the war inside you; the need to fight back; the 'I can't take this' feeling. You then need to move away from the source of violence where possible. A healthy self-esteem can go a long way in helping you let go of slights and offences.

People go through different experiences that informs subsequent behaviour. If you have been a victim of violence in the past, you may have a tendency to show violent behaviour.

If you notice that you show violence to other people, it is important to identify the root cause of your behaviour.

You do not have to be a victim of violence to show violence, if you have also witnessed or experienced abuse, you might have increased tendency to display interpersonal violence.

Speaking to someone about your experience, and getting some counselling may help you overcome the effects of negative experiences.

Counselling explores the basis of your experiences as a child or while growing up, and looks into why you may exhibit certain behaviours. It will also help you to look at practical ways to deal with this.

Young people sometimes feel as though counselling is too generalised and not helpful. This is not usually the case.

The good thing about speaking to someone is that counselling can be tailored towards your circumstances, experiences, and situation.

Knowing the right type of friends to associate with also helps with limiting the spread of interpersonal violence. Friends who make you better will most likely not get involved with violence.

Also making good use of the support systems around you can also help prevent interpersonal violence. Support systems such as those found in the school environment or at home; family and friends, vocational clubs, faith-based organisations and even your family doctor. Good support systems help engage young people in activities that foster positive relationships and interactions.

2

FORMING HEALTHY RELATIONSHIPS

Relationships are a very important part of our lives. Because you are a social being, you are bound to interact with people around you. This is simply how human beings are wired. Every day, we can either have a negative or positive impact on our relationships. It is important not to just form relationships but to have healthy ones.

The first thing to consider is knowing what it means to be in a healthy relationship. In a healthy relationship, you learn and grow. The person or people that you have relationships with also learn and grow as a result of their being associated with you. You want to be around people who hold you in high esteem, value you, and make you happy.

A good litmus test should be; Am I learning and growing in this relationship?

It is okay to disagree on matters but are you learning? Disagreements and issues usually arise in relationships but solving these issues and learning from disputes is a sign of a healthy relationship.

You do not always need to be right, nor do you have to win all arguments. Be careful if you are in a relationship of any kind where one person always seems to be right without respecting the other person's views.

Some young people find it challenging to form healthy, friendly relationships with their parents. The impression is that their parents do not care about them until they are going through difficulties or "misbehaving".

In many instances, no matter how old you are, if you make decisions that your parents don't agree with, this can cause conflict.

Let's take this dialogue as an example-

You say 'Dad, I need to attend a party at 8 pm tonight'.

Dad, 'Oh I see, how well are you familiar with the people you're going out with?'

You reply, 'Well daddy they are my school pals'.

Dad says, 'Do you know them well enough?' 'I don't think you should attend that party'. Such disagreements can lead to conflict. Realising that parents are more experienced and want the good of their children can enhance your forming and maintaining good relationships with them.

Healthy relationships with parents take conscious effort and time to create. Talking about issues that bother you, and listening to their concerns, even when you do not agree, will strengthen your relationship with them.

Building healthy relationships with people around you helps you feel less isolated. Feeling isolated can be frustrating, and is unhealthy in the long run.

If you have not built healthy, good relationships with the people around you, you can feel very lonely even with your immediate family present.

Loneliness or isolation can come from the experiences you had while growing up. You may also feel lonely if you lack confidence or you feel unworthy of attention from people close to you.

With this in mind it is also important to understand that we all have differences in our upbringing. The way we were brought up wires us and shapes our behaviour and attitude. Knowing this will make you feel less disappointed when people do not meet up to your expectations in relationships. Instead of feeling bad when people disappoint you, you may want to look for the good in each individual you relate with.

As a young person you might be finding it difficult to build healthy relationships. Here are some tips:

1. Be realistic with your expectations of people. We all have our strength and weaknesses. Learn to find and appreciate the good attributes of the people in your life.
2. Be yourself around your friends. It's easier and less stressful to be who you are in a healthy relationship.
3. Whenever you have a disagreement, try to cool off your emotions before talking.
4. Growth within a relationship can sometimes bring some discomfort. Prepare your mind for changes in your relationship. This will help with your emotions when you experience change.
5. Show kindness and respect.
6. Set boundaries and have the ability to say no when needed.

3

WHEN PARENTS DON'T DO RIGHT

The man was in his forties. He was in a hospital bed with tubes coming out of his chest and nose, blood dripping from a gash on the side of his head. The doctor walked into the room and told him 'You have just had an accident'…

'Really?', he replied as he felt a mixture of panic and deep pain in his head. 'So is this the end?' He tried to speak…

Then the flashback came …. A mental picture of him at the age of four, his Dad looking fierce and angry in a completely drunken state, hitting his mother across the back with a heavy metal chain. As his Mum screamed, he screamed out from his hospital bed … 'Help me! Please help me!'

This was the first time in 40 years that he would experience a flash back to his childhood trauma. He carried that experience in his subconscious for years, unaware. It came out when he was on the thin line between life and death.

You might get disappointed in relationships with your friends, an ex-boyfriend or girlfriend, or your siblings but emotional pain caused by parents often runs deeper and hurts worse.

A lot of young people have either experienced or witnessed violence, separation or divorce of parents, parental alcoholism/drug addiction and other traumatic childhood events. If all you saw while you were growing up was a lot of emotional, physical, verbal or sexual abuse, you are not alone. If in the process of your growing up you wished you experienced more of your mother's love or you wished your dad had treated your mum better than he did, your feelings and emotions are valid. If you have been a victim of childhood trauma brought about by your parents, it might affect your view about life or relationships as you form your own. This happens unconsciously and is not your fault. A lot of young people vividly remember landmarks of a major family breakdown and these memories linger on. You need to realise that it is normal for you to feel this way.

These experiences cause deep emotional wounds from which healing can be challenging. These wounds can cause pain in the process of trying to form your own healthy relationship with your siblings, your parents, your friends, your co-workers and when the time comes, with your spouse.

More so, if emotional wounds do not heal over time, this could lead to long-standing physical illnesses which can be difficult to treat or cure.

Understand that this is a process that can be likened to a journey. Just as it takes time for any physical wound to heal, healing from emotional wounds also takes time.

Your life is different, you are not the same as your parents and you can form healthy relationships by tending and caring for those wounds.

Not only can you develop and build relationships with those around you but you can do the same with your parents who have disappointed you.

Clearing your mind from all past wounds and hatred is a good place to start to form healthy relationships.

Meditations, prayers, affirmations can help the process of changing the way you think about yourself and your relationships with your parents.

Meditation is a practice which involves training your awareness and attention to achieve a mentally and emotionally clear state.

A popular example is the breathing technique during which you give attention to your breathing.

Prayers means you submit to a higher power to help you deal with issues you do not find easy to let go of. Having some few minutes set aside in the morning to pray is usually helpful.

Affirmation is having a vision of where you want to be and do and saying it loud to yourself. With time this sinks into your subconscious and you start to live in that vision.

All these lead to the beginning of forgiving and forging a new kind of relationship.

Forgiveness means you consciously let go of feelings of annoyance toward someone who has hurt you.

It does not mean you have forgotten, neither does it mean you are giving reasons for their actions. It can be difficult to forgive but it is a major step to breaking free. It has been found that the act of forgiveness keeps you healthy, helps low mood and reduces your anxiety and stress levels.

If possible, you might want to reach out to your parents let them know that you've forgiven them.

4

HANDLING A BREAKUP WITHOUT A BREAKDOWN

As a young person, you experiment with relationships. *This is part of the journey in making you an adult with healthy relationships.*

Relationships involving young people break up easily and it is only normal because you or your partner may not be emotionally ready for the long term commitment that it takes to sustain a relationship.

I have come across young people who become depressed after going through a breakup. It is normal to feel this way if you have gone through, or are going through a breakup. You probably felt very good about this relationship. You thought you would live happily ever after. But sometime breakups happen and you need time to heal.

It does not matter if you are a boy or a girl; it is understandable to feel disappointed, rejected and down.

When relationships break down, seeing it as a learning process can help you to heal better.

Open up to trusted loved ones for emotional and moral support to help you.

After a break up, you might feel as though you're not good enough which is why it happened. This is not true. Realise you're good and worthy and everyone is just in the process of becoming better. Have a deep think, reason and help yourself understand why the relationship broke up. Relationships break up for a reason and many times it is better that it happened sooner rather than later. In long-term relationships where you have invested a lot into it over time, having a breakup could negatively affect either of the parties involved.

The period of feeling down after a breakup should not last long. Give yourself time and space to feel this way. Do not think you are abnormal to have these feelings. The good thing is that these feelings pass with time. It might be difficult but this is a time to relax, become more confident and get friendly with other people.

This is the time to allow yourself to heal, pick up a hobby and develop yourself. Develop into a new you.

Engaging yourself with things you enjoy can help you during this period. What are the things you enjoy doing? This is the time to plunge into those things. When you engage in activities that keep you busy, you find it easier to put things behind you and start a new life.

5

BULLYING

Bullying occurs when someone uses some form of power over you to hurt you over and over again.

Bullying is currently a major issue in young people. It is so common that you too probably have been bullied.

Bullying can be physical or emotional. With emotional bullying, the bully tries to make you feel that they have power over you by making you feel hurt or frightened.

Why do young people get involved with bullying? What causes bullying? Most young people who engage in bullying experienced a lot of issues while growing up or are currently experiencing them at home.

The first step is to understand why people engage in bullying. They might do so in order to make you feel less important. Some people do not feel they have power or popularity so they try to attain these through negative means. Bullies usually have low self-esteem and as a result may resort to attention seeking behaviour.

Who are those at high risk of being bullied?

Bullies usually look for vulnerable people to bully. *Vulnerability in the sense of being weak and easily hurt physically or emotionally.* This might manifest as being unable to speak up for yourself, inability to make decisions or physical inequality with your peers.

When you are a victim of bullying, understanding why people engage in bullying can help you deal with it in a positive way.

If you are being bullied, the first step is to consciously put yourself in a superior position to your bully. This is called a positive response. This is where your self-esteem comes in, and you deliberately tell yourself that you are not the picture being painted by the bully.

Responding to bullying in a negative way by retaliating will only fuel the bullying process. Trying to get back at them can make your bully identify your sensitive spots (those issues that get you easily irritated). They might then use these against you in the future.

It is important to note that bullying usually escalates, worsening with each episode.

Trying to regain your confidence after experiencing bullying might be hard. Here are tips on what to do after you have been bullied:

1. Accept that it is normal to experience stress, anxiety or low mood after being bullied.
2. Talk to trusted people like your parents, teachers, friends, or counsellors about how you feel. Not letting out your feelings might create increased anxiety and stress.
3. Try to actively engage in living a healthy lifestyle –good nutrition, exercise and adequate sleep.
4. Practice journal writing. Write about issues bothering you at the moment. Write about things to be grateful for. This can help you recover after a period of being bullied.

On the flip side, what if you are the bully?

Young people might engage in bullying because they need to feel that they are in control, they want to gain popularity. They may also be modelling abuse that they encountered while growing up. In addition, a person with low self-esteem may find it easy to bully others.

If you find yourself bullying others, you may need to speak to someone (a counsellor) who might be able to help. Counsellors can help you understand why you behave the way you do and explore practical ways to help you out.

JOURNALING ON RELATIONSHIPS

1. What are the 10 supportive systems available to me as a young adult?

2. What are the practical ways to help me deal with bullying?

3. Do I have a healthy relationship with my parents or loved ones?

4. What do I like about my closest friend?

5. Why am I in a boyfriend-girlfriend relationship at the moment?

PART THREE
MENTAL HEALTH

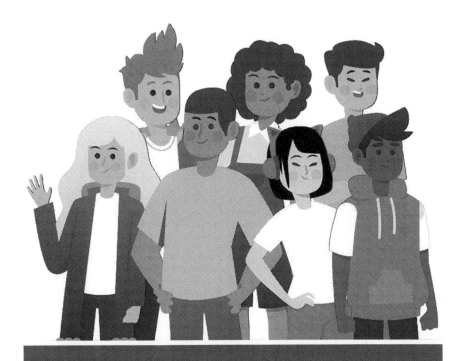

1

OVERCOMING ANXIETY AND STRESS

Stress is a state of mental or emotional strain or tension resulting from adverse or very demanding circumstances. We all feel stress from time to time.

Anxiety is a feeling of worry, nervousness, or unease, typically about an imminent event or something with an uncertain outcome. Being anxious is also quite common.

Anxiety as a psychiatric condition is a nervous disorder characterised by a state of excessive uneasiness and apprehension, typically with compulsive behaviour or panic attacks. This type is extreme and usually requires the care of a psychiatrist.

Stress and anxiety results when we don't have the emotional resources to cope with whatever adverse circumstances we might be facing.

There are many causes of stress. Examples range from taking exams to a death in the family. It is important to develop specific skills and mechanisms for coping with stress. It would be unrealistic to think that you will never have any stress.

Unhealthy coping mechanisms if used in dealing with normal stress can lead to anxiety and fear.

Healthy ways of coping with stress include:

1. Breathing exercises.
2. Frequent mental breaks.
3. Exercise including dancing.
4. Listening to inspiring music.
5. Focusing on the positive.
6. Prayer and meditation.
7. Positive affirmations.
8. Talking to supportive friends.
9. Talking walks in nature.
10. Being outside in the sun.
11. Making time for fun in your daily life.
12. Talking to your therapist or doctor.
13. Having social connections.
14. Doing activities that make you feel happy on a daily basis.
15. Processing, rather than avoiding negative emotions.

A WORD ON EXAM STRESS

Exams are a normal part of life for many young people in secondary school and university. You will typically need to pass exams to get to a new level, a new class, or to gain a degree. In order to minimise exam stress you need to develop a study plan that allows you to prepare for your upcoming exams and tests in small increments. Trying to study all the material the night before a test can create more anxiety and fear.

Eating healthy in order keep your blood sugar levels steady is important. This will prevent sudden lowering of your blood sugar and help keep a steady supply of energy to your brain. Using some of the coping mechanisms mentioned above can help calm your mind. If you suffer from crippling test anxiety that prevents you from taking or passing exams, talk to your doctor to explore what your options are.

2

SELF-ESTEEM

Self-esteem is defined as: *'One's attitude towards oneself or one's opinion or evaluation of oneself, which may be positive (favourable or high), neutral, or negative (unfavourable or low)'.*

Self-esteem is usually used to describe how you think and feel about yourself. Self-esteem starts from building a strong relationship with your body and mind. Self-esteem is that nurturing aspect you feel with yourself.

Everyone has a relationship with their body and mind and you have to decide what sort of relationship you would like to build with yourself.

At some stage in your life, usually as you reach adolescence, you begin to have a more conscious nature of yourself. The quality of that relationship will either lead to low or high self-esteem.

Some effects of negative or low self-esteem are:

1. Self-hate: Not liking your looks, your speech, and other things that make you, you.
2. Feelings of inadequacy.
3. Excessive people pleasing.

It takes conscious effort to tell and remind yourself who you really are and to not to be defined by the relationships you experienced while growing up.

How do I build positive self-esteem?

If you have been affected by negative experiences, it takes a conscious effort to remind yourself of your worth.

Building positive self-esteem starts with investing in your body and mind. You need a healthy lifestyle; good sleep, adequate exercise, a good diet and healthy relationships.

A healthy diet nourishes your body. Generally a healthy diet in simple terms for young people is a diet rich in plant-based foods. It's okay to start trying vegetables and fruit in your diet.

Good sleep means you have good quality of sleep away from noise and distractions.

You feel revived and energetic in the morning.

Why do I need to build positive self-esteem?

Positive self-esteem means you believe you can overcome any challenge. It makes you believe in yourself.

Having high self-esteem means you do not demean your behaviours, your values, the way you look or the way you feel.

Building positive self-esteem will go a long way in helping you face any challenging issues that may be bound to happen through as you journey through life.

3

LOW MOOD AND DEPRESSION

Being depressed is a situation in which in addition to your feeling low in mood, you also lose interest in the things you typically enjoy. When you feel low in mood you may notice other changes in your thinking and in your actions. You might notice some other symptoms such as lack of concentration or attention, not eating or sleeping well, not thinking about the future, low self-esteem, lack of self-confidence, low energy and constantly feeling guilty.

Some young people might actually experience physical symptoms such as headaches, body aches, and stomach aches.

The most serious of them all is the thought of ending one's life.

Mood swings are very common in young people because of hormonal changes. This feeling can sometimes be normal and does not always mean that you have a depressed mood.

It is important to know that there might be some differences in symptoms of depression between adults and young people.

Adults may experience sleep problems, sadness and withdrawal when they feel depressed while young people will generally express their feelings through anger and irritability.

Some young adults have depression which continues right into adulthood and can significantly affect their lives.

There are a number of reasons why you might feel depressed.

This might be because someone in your family has a history of depression, or other mental health problems.

You might experience family or social life happenings such as a separation between mum and dad, loss of a loved one, or one or both your parents losing their job(s) and even losing a home.

Unpleasant things might have happened to you in the past such as physical, emotional, or sexual abuse. You might also have experienced bullying or neglect. You might have depression if you have been using alcohol or drugs. If you have a long-term illness you might experience depression or depressive episodes.

Knowing what to do when you have low mood and depression is important because if this is not taken care of, it can lead to several other problems such as poor school or work performance. Paradoxically, depression can lead to drugs and alcohol abuse or difficulty with making and keeping friends.

The first step is realising that there are different degrees of severity of depression.

- Mild depression where a person experiences symptoms which may interfere with your day-to-day activities. It can result in anger, loss of interest in activities you enjoy, difficulties with concentration, and sleep disturbances.

- Moderate depression which can present with additional symptoms such as feeling of worthlessness, self-esteem and excessive worry and anxiety. You will most likely experience symptoms associated with mild depression.

- Severe Depression where symptoms listed for mild or moderate depression are usually more pronounced and becomes easily noticeable to external persons. You might have the following— hallucinations, which means seeing or hearing things which others are not experiencing; delusions which consists of strong unshakeable beliefs that are not actually true. Self-harm or suicidal feelings can also be associated with severe depression.

It is important to identify where you're struggling and the root cause of why you may be depressed. Identifying the root cause for your low mood will help you to think of practical ways to deal with this.

You also need to understand that it is not unusual to feel this way if especially if you have experienced certain life issues.

A lot of young people I see in my practice say things like 'I have gone through low mood and anxiety for quite a while, I thought that I could deal with this on my own' or they say 'I don't feel like talking or speaking to anyone'.

Realise that you cannot deal with this on your own. You need help and the first step is knowing that you need to speak to, or see a professional.

If you cannot speak to your Parents or family members, there are different services to help you. These include mental health clinics, youth outreach services, school-based early intervention programmes, young peoples' counselling services or your family doctor.

Your doctor may want to be sure that there are no other medical causes for why you feel this way. They may arrange for some blood tests such as checking for your iron levels and levels of some key vitamins such as Vitamin B and D. Iron and vitamin deficiencies have been linked to mental health.

Depending on what your doctor finds, you might be prescribed therapy and/or antidepressants.

Remember, maintaining a healthy lifestyle through exercise, good diet, adequate sleep and positive relationships will help your mental health in the long run.

4

SOCIAL MEDIA

Social media helps us create and share information, share ideas and express ourselves with others around us. We are social beings and as a young person you feel the need to connect, to interact, to belong and to make your presence known.

More than ever, you want to be accepted and approved. Social media has a lot of advantages —you can catch up with friends and family all over the world. You can learn and share bright ideas with other people of like minds. You can also make new friends. As a technological invention, social media is and has helped solve a lot of problems, but the fact remains that there is a major side effect; A tendency to get addicted.

There are other notable downsides. Social media has discouraged face to face interaction and interaction with nature. Too much of it can increase anxiety, low mood and loneliness.

You may find that what is meant to make you more connected with friends and family can produce a negative effect and ends up making you feel isolated.

Friends, families, acquaintances, and influencers all portray their best appearances on social media. This might make you feel less important, thinking you're not meeting up to a certain standard.

In the light of the coronavirus pandemic, communicating through social media has become even more critical for keeping up with family and friends, but it is very important that there is a balance in all of this.

What can you do if you find that you engage too much with social media?

- Disconnect: Try to turn off your personal phone during work, meal, recreational activities, sleep, when friends are visiting.
- Adjust: Create settings on each social media app to turn off (and on) at certain times.
- Set it: Dedicate set times to use social media per day.
- Time it: Use a timer to help you keep account of how much time you spend on social media.

This might be difficult at first but you find that you get used to it with time.

5

DRUGS, ALCOHOL AND TOBACCO USE

Drugs and alcohol contain powerful brain stimulating chemicals. These stimulants may create good feelings initially but these effects unfortunately do not last long. People take more drugs and alcohol in order to experience the good feelings again. This can set up a vicious cycle of addiction and addictive behaviours.

Why do young people go into drugs and alcohol use?

There are lots of reasons

Boredom and peer pressure are among the top reasons for young people experimenting with alcohol and drugs.

A lot of young people do not think of the addictive nature of drugs and alcohol especially when trying it out the first time.

Taking a step back to think about the after-effects can help you stay away from drugs and alcohol.

Drugs and alcohol can cause a lot of negative effects:

1. They can affects your self-esteem and cause a feeling of emptiness after the effects of the drugs ("the high") have worn off.
2. They can also lead to feelings of guilt and shame that result from the knowledge that these substances are not good for your body or your mind. Feelings of guilt also lead to self-isolation which in turn can increase your use of drugs and/or alcohol.
3. They can affect your ability to make correct decisions both in the short term and on the long run.
4. Alcohol-related vehicle crashes leading to physical injuries are a direct result of involvement with alcohol and drugs. These physical injuries can be life-changing. Alcohol and drug use can also cause problems with normal growth or sexual development.
5. Increased incidence of mental health problems.
6. Increased risk of using drugs and alcohol into adulthood due to their addictive nature.

More importantly they can have other long-term effects on your health farther in the future.

A lot of young people are being tempted to go into drugs and alcohol by peer pressure.

When you are faced such a dilemma, or being exposed to drugs, consciously taking a step back to think of the immediate effects will help you to make the right decisions. You can also take note of following tips:

1) Staying focused on the reasons why you should keep away from drugs and alcohol is always helpful.

2) Paying attention to your circle of friends.

If you have a friend who is involved in drugs and alcohol, you are more likely to be influenced.

3) Developing new hobbies.

Since boredom is a major reason for young people to go into drugs and alcohol, new hobbies can help keep young people occupied.

4) Thinking through and discussing with family practical ways to deal with peer pressure by turning down offers of drugs or alcohol.

If you are involved with drug and alcohol, get professional help from your doctor. Speak to a counsellor who can also direct you to appropriate services.

JOURNALING ON MENTAL HEALTH

1. What 5 things do I love about myself?

2. Name 5 compliments people have ever made to me?

3. What is my personal view about my exams and studies?

4. Name 5 areas which I readily stress about?

5. How do I think I can deal with these stresses?

PART FOUR
A HEALTHY LIFESTYLE

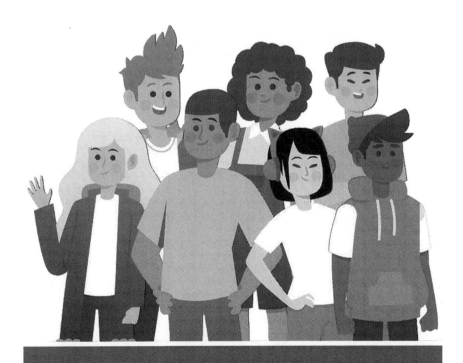

1

YOU ARE WHAT YOU EAT!

You are what you eat is a common saying.

Hippocrates once said: "Let food be thy medicine, and let medicine be thy food."

The times I felt the best about myself was when I had fruits and vegetables as a large portion of my diet. It was amazing to feel so good in my body soon after eating. More than ever, we need to be more conscious about what we eat and drink because we are now more aware of the impact on our bodies.

Food is a big issue! Especially with a lot of information on TV, the internet, in our community, and coming from family and friends about diet: what you should eat, how you should cook and what recipes to make and so on. Generally the less processed the food is, the healthier it is.

Healthy eating involves the act of conscious eating. Know that I am also working on this myself.

To make it simple; a diet that has more fruit and vegetables is a good place to start.

Think about what kind of fruits and vegetables you enjoy eating. Make it fill half your plate at every meal then fill the other portion of your plate with other food groups.

Starting with something simple—ensuring you have 5 portions of fruit and vegetables a day and gradually making small changes will go a long way. You can get a log book to help you with this.

There is an important connection between what you eat and the way you feel. There are studies to show that your diet can help prevent and address mental health problems.

A diet that is generally rich in fruits and vegetables, and supplemented with fish oil has been proven to help improve low mood. They do this by releasing feel good chemicals called serotonin and dopamine which might help regulate your sleep and improve your mood.

While this is not a book about diets, recognize that diets such as the Mediterranean diet can be part of healthy eating. Diets like this consists mostly of plant based foods especially vegetables, fruits, legumes, and fats such as olive oil. They allow for a limited amount of dairy, fish and meat.

Important vitamins like Vitamin B12 and Vitamin D can be found in a balanced diet, and can help boost your mental health. Vitamin B12 is largely related to animal sources such as fish, meat, eggs, poultry and dairy products. Other ways of getting vitamin B12, include Vitamin B12 fortified foods such as cereals or B12 supplements sold in chemists. Healthy fats and Omega 3 fatty acids can be found in oily fish, walnut oil and flax seed. If you are vegetarian or a vegan, you might get your Vitamin B12 from foods like flaxseeds and walnuts.

2

Sleep should be healthy. Healthy sleep is one that refreshes us.

It is said that teens need eight to ten hours of sleep while young adults need about seven to nine hours. After a good night's sleep, you should feel restored, energetic and prepared for a new day. Problems with sleep in young people are not that common unless you are prone to night terrors, nightmares.

The process of falling asleep starts from a short period of 20- 30 minutes after which you go into a long period of deep sleep known as slow wave sleep. Slow wave sleep is usually deep and refreshing. If your slow wave sleep is interrupted, you might not feel refreshed in the morning. The REM (Rapid Eye Movement) stage of sleep involves dreaming.

Lack of refreshing sleep is a common complaint among young people. The good thing is that just by taking some simple measures, you can improve your sleep pattern.

Have a set time for going to bed each night. This is because when you have a set time, your mind reminds your body that you need to go to bed. It is said that it takes about three weeks to turn a practice into a habit.

Try putting gadgets off for about 1 hour before your set bedtime. Social gadgets such as phones, and iPads can also be a distraction. When you are focused on a light source and pictures from these gadgets before bedtime, your mind tells your body that you still need to be active. You may then find it more difficult to switch from a screen mode where you are attentive and awake to the restful mode required for having a good night's sleep.

For young people drinking some warm milk can help. Milk contains an important nutrient called tryptophan. Tryptophan helps the brain and gut produce chemicals called serotonin and melatonin which help you relax and feel good.

3

EXERCISE

When you think about exercise what runs through your mind?

You think you already exercise a lot as your day is filled with activities.

I hear a lot people say, I work hard and that is a form of exercise because I am never still, particularly at work.

Exercise is not the same as physical activity.

Exercise involves organized, purposeful movements which results in increased heart rate; feeling your heart pumping and hearing yourself breathe faster.

Physical activity is about getting involving in activities beyond your baseline. It means you're using more energy than you normally use while in a sedentary state.

The time duration is also very important.

20 minutes seven days a week, or 30 minutes five days a week is a good duration for an adequate amount of exercise.

Exercise makes your heart pump (faster), which helps oxygen get delivered more briskly to your brain and body. This makes you feel refreshed and energetic in the long run. Exercise can strengthen the muscles and make you feel refreshed.

When a part of your body receives less oxygen it tends to ache after a while. Aches and pains can improve with exercise.

It might be difficult to exercise as a young person but here are some practical ways to get moving.

The first attitude is to bear in mind is about finding time and to remember that all movement counts.

- If you school nearby, rather than taking a bus to school, try jogging and brisk walking.
- Running upstairs, using the stairs instead of an elevator, choosing to do some yard work all gives an opportunity to exercise.
- You could join a sports club and use this opportunity to engage in healthy challenges and exercise sessions.

Taking care of your mental health can also encourage you to exercise. If you feel depressed, you are less likely to exercise.

Your exercise does not have to be all in one go but finding activities that will add up to your 30 minutes a day is okay.

At the end of each day, ask yourself how many minutes of exercise you have been able to achieve. A log book can help with this.

4

MEDITATION

Don't close the book yet! Young people do not always think about meditation. They think it is old people's stuff.

There are different forms of meditation. While on this topic, we will discuss suitable forms for young people.

Meditation is a practice where you use a technique such as simple breathing or focusing your mind on a particular image or object to train your attention and awareness.

When you constantly train your awareness, your emotions become more stable and your mental health improves.

Meditation comes in different forms and there are lots of studies on the benefits of meditation. Starting with something as simple as focusing on your breathing and allowing yourself feel the change in your body is a great way to start. As a young person, you might just focus on breathing techniques daily for a few minutes.

This reminds me of a story of a lady who always woke up at 5:30 every morning to meditate. Now you don't have to wake up at 5:30 am to do this. Just choose a time that is suitable for you.

Back to the story, this lady practiced meditation every morning and then decided she should [could also] get the children involved. In the process of doing this over weeks, her daughter confessed that she had thoughts of committing suicide and had kept it a secret for a long time. Through meditation, the daughter volunteered this information and was able to get the necessary help and support from her parents.

It is known that the process of meditation allows you to handle your emotions, it is calming to your body and soul.

Meditation helps health and happiness.

Another facet to meditation is prayer. Prayer means that you are submitting yourself to God; a higher Being who has power to help you with those things beyond your control. There are many happenings beyond our control. A recent example would be the coronavirus pandemic that led to the whole world shutting down. In this case, knowing that God has the world in His hands allows you to turn over situations completely over to Him. Research has been done on the benefits of prayer. It has been shown to calm one's nerves, diminishing your fight or flight response. It has also been found to make people less reactive to negative emotions. And makes us less angry.

Positive Confessions means speaking out loud to yourself, the positive experiences you want to bring into your life. Some people call these positive confessions, affirmations.

You can write your positive confessions in a journal and read them to yourself for about 2-3 minutes every morning.

You might want to practice what I call 'creating your day'. In this practice, you visualise how you want your day to be. Visualising your anticipated actions from the start of the day helps you plan your day.

Your day might not fall in perfectly with what you imagined, but trying to figure out what you want to do in the course of the day would put you back on track. It helps you to get more focused and ready for a new day. It gives you the energy you need to live the day.

5

HOBBIES

What is a hobby?

A hobby is an activity done regularly in one's leisure time for pleasure.

Hobbies can be easy or difficult but you'll usually derive pleasure from doing it.

Taking up a hobby is a great way to get you busy and help you feel more balanced.

The good thing about taking on a hobby is that you can turn this into a source of income as you start your working life.

You have this gift over the years, you are more experienced and you have more to offer.

You can develop competency in your hobbies to the point that they can add value to others, and become a stream/source of income.

What is your passion?

Things you can do or talk about even when woken up from your sleep are likely the things that you have a passion or a flair for.

I have a passion for writing and I decided to develop this further by writing a book.

I remember when I was in junior school, I would write plays and stories in a notebook and give them to my classmates to read. They always enjoyed them. As I moved through secondary school and on to medical school, I got distracted from my passion for writing.

I later found that having a passion in something other than your main career can make you feel more balanced, more focused and help your mental health in the long run. So I revived my passion for the written word.

Can you act, sing, write, cook...the list goes on and on.

You can start by making a list of five things that naturally come to you and five areas that you wish to learn more about.

Can you learn more about your hobby? Are there books written about your current hobby? Are there people who know more about your hobby who you can learn from? There are books for almost any area you would like to develop yourself. A good one is the "Dummies series".

If you know someone or people who have excelled in an area you are passionate about, then learn from them. Buy their books, listen to them online if available, watch their videos.

You can simply search in Google names of people who have excelled in –'Your field'.

Are there any support systems in your area that can help you develop your hobby? In my local community, there are programmes done yearly for different crafts and hobbies.

You can also learn a hobby even it is not what you are naturally talented to do.

All you need is to dedicate at least one hour a week to focus attention on your hobby.

You might not be all perfect but starting out is good.

You never know how lucrative this might turn out to be!

JOURNALING FOR
HEALTHY LIFESTYLE

1. What areas of my lifestyle do I need to work on?

2. How do I intend to work on these in the next three to six months?

3. How likely am I to achieve any goals set in these areas in the next three to six months?

4. What positive changes have I noticed about my lifestyle and habits?

PART FIVE
COMMON MEDICAL CONDITIONS

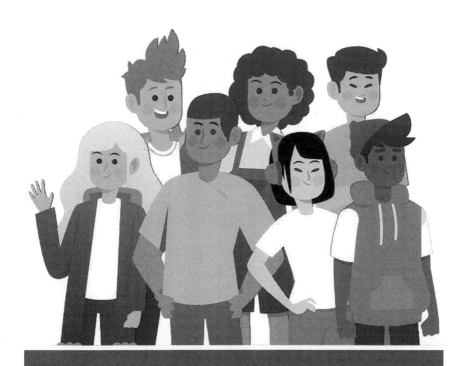

1

EATING DISORDERS

The young lady sitting on the hospital bed looked very thin and pale. The dinner lady brought in some food. She looked at the food in disgust. Her Mother stood by her side, urging her to eat.

The doctor came around the bed – Her Mum told the doctor the daughter had developed this poor relationship with food since starting college. She would not eat meat, fish or dairy and she would skip meals. She kept a weighing scale underneath her bed which she used every morning and evening. She also had a large full size mirror that she continually gazed into after bathing every morning.

The problem began with her giving excuses about being too busy to eat, then escalated to missing family dinners. She soon began to feel weak and started to miss her periods.

The doctor gently reassured her Mum that she would be fine but this it would take a gradual process of love, support, and joint care from the hospital and her family.

Eating disorders are serious conditions related to persistent eating behaviours that negatively impact your health, your emotions and your ability to function in important areas of life. The most common eating disorders are anorexia nervosa, bulimia nervosa and binge eating disorder.

Eating disorders cannot be ignored due to the importance people attach to weight loss and looking good. A lot of magazines, social media and the society talk about how to lose weight, go on diets, and improve our body shape.

Young people now associate their self-esteem with a thin body.

Actors, models and other celebrities often contribute to this narrative by altering their pictures to look slimmer (Photoshopping); going on extreme diets, endorsing questionable diet pills, and fat shaming others.

If you find that you have lost interest in food, you may have an eating disorder. You may feel as if you are too thin because you are not eating enough.

Low energy, tiredness, weakness, and feeling mentally slow can be symptoms of an eating disorder.

You might have binge eating disorder if you experience a loss of control and overeat on a regular basis.

Sometimes anxiety and low mood due to how you feel about your body image can lead to problems with eating. You might be a picky eater. You might find it difficult to stop eating and sometimes feel the urge to eat constantly. This can lead to weight gain.

Eating disorders might be difficult to deal with especially if you are trying to seek solutions on your own.

There are some measures that you can take to manage eating disorders. Meal planning and family involvement are some of the ways to help young people with eating disorders. Meal planning is when you prepare your meals in a way that ensures you get the necessary nutrients to help you get better physically as well as improve your mental health while you recover from an eating disorder. Meal planning will also help you to make healthy food choices.

You need to keep track of how you feel mentally. Avoid long periods of not eating. Not eating for about 4 hours brings hunger pangs which make you eat more with your next meal.

Avoid Yo-yo dieting. Yo-yo dieting is used to describe a cycle of weight loss and weight gain. It is much better to maintain a stable weight over a period of time. This can be done by trying to lose weight slowly and in a most convenient way.

When you go on fad diets, using fat burners or going on replacement shakes, you lose weight drastically. Once you slip back into old eating habits you gain the weight back again and even more. This cycle can affect your mental health in a most negative way and make you more prone to eating disorders.

There are habits that tend to make us gain weight or make weight loss a bit more difficult.

Here are some of them:

1. Eating while watching TV.
2. Not getting enough Sleep.
3. Skipping Breakfast.
4. Eating too many processed or sugary foods.
5. Not drinking enough water.
6. Eating too quickly.
7. Eating from large plates.
8. Not eating enough fibre or protein.

9. Not having set eating times.
10. Having too much salad dressing.

Try to focus on your health while you seek help. Focusing on how to get rid of many of these habits will be more helpful in maintaining a steady, and healthy weight for you.

Doctors will work with mental health professionals to treat and provide support if you have an eating disorder. Nutritionists, dieticians, social workers and mental health professionals work as team during your care. There are also physical problems that tends to accompany eating disorders. You need to ensure you see a doctor who can arrange other tests to be sure you're not lacking in any vitamins. You might need a supplements or vitamins while undergoing treatment for eating disorders.

2

HEADACHES

Headache is a term used to describe pain felt in the head.

It is a very common symptom across all age groups. A young person at one time or the other would have complained about a headache. A headache that lasts for a prolonged time can cause worry and anxiety. A young man I saw while I was a junior doctor came in with headaches that he had had for several months. The headache was mild and would come on at a certain time each day. He was so concerned that he had a brain tumour although he did not have other signs of one.

There are several types of headache and some forms are more common in younger adults. Migraines and tension headaches are some of these common types of headache.

MIGRAINES:

People with migraines have their headache occurring intermittently. They could occur on a monthly, weekly or daily basis. They typically last about four to seventy two hours if left untreated. The headache is usually one sided. This pain is usually described as excruciating. Some may experience problems with their vision such as flashing lights or develop weakness or sensation problems with their limbs during their migraines. You may feel sick or have vomiting with your migraine. Migraines may have a familial predisposition.

We know that there are possible triggers for migraine attacks and trying to avoid your known triggers can go a long way to control your migraine. Having a headache diary will also help you to keep track of what you think the triggers are and then try to avoid them. Triggers include foods such as dairy, cheese, chocolate, and alcohol. Stress, being tired or hungry, exercise, contraceptive pills containing oestrogen, are some other non-food triggers.

Pills are generally used to treat or to prevent migraines. If you are prone to having a lot of migraines, your doctor might decide to prescribe medications to help prevent migraines rather than treating them.

TENSION HEADACHES

Tension headaches are another common type of headaches.

They are usually milder than migraines and can typically last from 30 minutes to about 7 days in some prolonged cases.

They can be one-sided or felt all over the head but it is typically felt as a tight band around the head. It often spreads to or starts from the neck. A tension headache is often caused by stress, anxiety or mood changes such as depression.

When you're feeling stressed, the neck muscles can go into spasm or tension which can then cause a tension headache.

With these headaches, you do not usually have the typical symptoms that you might get with a migraine headache like feeling sick, or problems with your vision or feeling generally unwell. Because a tension headache is related to stress and anxiety things like regular exercise, meditation and talking therapy can be used to treat it. Medications can also be used if any of the simple measures explained above are not helping.

Headaches can sometimes impact on your mood as they are unpleasant. This can also create anxiety and stress causing a vicious cycle. Remember, keeping a diary and noting the pattern of headache can help you when talking about your symptoms with your doctor.

3

An allergy is an immune system response to a foreign substance that's not typically harmful to your body. These foreign substances are called allergens. Allergies as a condition are quite common.

I recollect how prone I was as a teenager to having a sore throat, a runny nose, along with coughing and sneezing. I soon outgrew this when I got into high school. Looking back, I am not sure if I had allergies then. The good thing is that I no longer have these symptoms often.

Most people with allergies most likely have had symptoms since their childhood. Some may get better as they grow older while some keep having many symptoms well into adulthood.

Allergies are caused by your body fighting against what is normally considered to be harmless. A lot of other conditions such as irritable bowel and intolerance to certain foods might mimic allergies.

Allergies can have different symptoms ranging from bowel symptoms such as tummy pain, loose stools or constipation, feeling sick or vomiting. You can also develop skin problems such as skin rashes. Other symptoms include cough, runny nose, stuffy nose and sneezing. Some severe forms of allergy can cause lip or mouth swelling, tongue swelling, difficulty breathing, or a rattling sound in the chest.

You can be allergic to a number of things such as food, house dust mites, pets, or dander.

WHAT YOU DO IF YOU THINK YOU HAVE AN ALLERGY?

If you ever develop lip, mouth or tongue swelling, difficulty breathing or rattling in your chest please seek emergency help straight away.

Keeping a diary can also help you to find out if you are allergic to certain types of foods or substances. It is important to avoid any foods or substances you think you may be allergic to. Symptoms of allergies can sometimes impact your mood. They can cause sleep disturbances. Thinking that you have an allergy makes you worry and can also affect your day-to-day activities. It may become necessary to seek help if you feel this way.

Know that you're not alone and that help is available for your allergies.

Use of tablets called antihistamines can reduce the body's production of chemicals responsible for your allergy symptoms.

4

PERIOD PROBLEMS

Period problems range from heavy periods painful periods or spotting. They are very common especially among young people. However they can become problematic, when they start to affect your day-to-day life.

When I was in secondary school there was a girl who would always miss her classes during her periods. She was almost bed-bound, needing painkillers like ibuprofen and paracetamol for the entire duration of her period.

No one needed to inform us that she was having her periods as we knew she would always miss classes without fail during that time.

It may be a nightmare trying to figure out why your periods are heavy or painful or irregular,

Period cramps can happen when the muscular part of your womb tightens up. Prostaglandin, a chemical made by the uterus causes the muscles of the womb to tighten and relax causing period cramps. These normally last for a few days but can last longer in some girls.

Period pains can be severe enough to affect school, work or day-to-day activities.

Your period pains can cause you greater anxiety, they may make you more emotional and you might begin to feel guilty for being a young woman. All of the anxiety and pain experienced might make you think doctor would not be able to help you.

The good thing is that there is help for your period pains.

Painkillers like paracetamol and ibuprofen can help. This helps in about seventy percent of people.

Some simple measures you can take at home to help you with period cramps include:

1. Taking a warm bath or shower: can help relieve pain and help you relax.
2. A belly massage can also help.
3. You may find putting a hot water bottle on your lower belly or lower back helpful.
4. Engaging in exercises such as lower back,hip and pelvic stretches.
5. Some people find meditation helpful.

Periods can also become very heavy such that they begin to affect your day-to-day life. Heavy periods are common in young people and they are not an indication that something is wrong.

The definition of heavy periods vary from person to person. Your periods are most likely heavy if you think they are. If you change your sanitary products very often, you most likely have heavy bleeds. When you see your doctor, they may want to find out if there are other reasons for your heavy bleeds. If there are no other causes for heavy bleeds, you might be put on tablets that will help make your periods lighter.

Periods can also become irregular, meaning you have difficulty in telling when your next periods will be.

On the average, periods last between two to seven days and occur every 28 days (monthly), approximately. If you have irregular periods, your doctor may put you on certain hormones in the form of pills that make your periods more regular. Keeping a period diary can help you keep track of your periods.

5

Acne are spots on the face which often occur in respond to hormone changes. You might be wondering why you are seeing unsightly spots on your face that were not there previously. Your skin makes a lot more hormones as you hit puberty and these hormones cause your skin to form more oil in the glands. Pores can then become blocked forming spots or acne. You can sometimes find these spots on your chest and back.

Acne is a common condition in young adults because a lot of hormones come into play at that stage. Acne is also common in both males and females.

If you have a severe form of acne, it could get inflamed and cause a lot of pain. Picking at your acne can cause a worsening of your spots. This causes your spots to get angry looking and can sometimes cause an infection.

Acne can have a psychological effect on you because you do not like the effects of these spots on the way you look.

The good thing is that there are measures you can take to help yourself. The first is understanding that your acne is not related to hygiene or to your diet. However, eating a generally healthy diet with lots of fruit and vegetables is good. Drinking lots of fluids is good—But water is best.

Avoiding oil-based make up is something else you can do. Glossy, oil -based make up might look better on your skin but may not be a good idea if you have acne since your face is already actively producing oils. Washing your face with a non-drying agent can help your acne. Use of pH-balanced facial washes and moisturisers can help.

Pills and topical creams can be prescribed for your acne.

For oily skin, gels are generally used but if you have dry skin you will want to use creams. Treating larger areas will usually require the use of lotions. Sometimes you might need to see a skin specialist (dermatologist) if medications prescribed by your doctor are not helping.

Avoiding stress is also important as stress can flare up acne.

Acne can sometimes cause problems with self-image making you feel ashamed. It can lead to low self-esteem.

A boy [I once consulted on] had terrible spots which affected his self-esteem, and he found it difficult to go out or make friends at school. He tried a lot of creams and lotions but did not get better.

He then tried to develop a conscious effort to love his skin and appearance even in that state. As time passed, and before he knew it, the acne cleared on its own.

Trying to accept yourself might be hard but knowing that this is a common condition and most often resolves with age is a good thing to bear in mind.

JOURNALING ON COMMON MEDICAL CONDITIONS

1. What do I know about my medical conditions?

2. What do I think is causing my conditions?

3. What practical ways can help me with my medical conditions?

4. In what ways are my medical conditions affecting my mood?

5. What am I most concerned about regarding my health?

CONCLUSION

This book has been written because we all need one another. We all go through challenges in life and young people are not exempted. Sharing knowledge, ideas and principles with others can go a long way to make us a better person.

Basic Lifestyle principles outlined in this book can help you become more well-rounded mentally and physically.

My hope is that by reading this book, you get to have a more positive outlook in facing many of the issues that may come your way. Identifying these issues is a first step. After reading this book, as a young person you will understand most of the common issues you might face. You will be able to look into how you can deal with these issues by building enough resilience. The tips included in this book are very handy and by picking this book to read, you show that you care about yourself mentally and physically. It shows you're taking responsibility for your mental and physical health. It gives you a sense of pride in yourself.

You most likely already have some knowledge about what you're going through for when you need to see a doctor. You may also have an idea of what questions you might be asked or questions you would want to ask if you need to speak to a counsellor. You might also have some first-hand knowledge about some of the issues discussed here. This book however, gives a well-rounded approach to both your mental and physical health.

I hope you continue to be well-rounded while maintaining resilience to achieve greater success in life.

I hope to hear from you.

'Your Family Doctor'

REFERENCES

1. Journal of Paediatric and Adolescent Gynaecology –Date Rape Among Adolescents and young Adults
2. 7 myths about the HPV Vaccine –HPV vaccine facts and the science behind them. Claire C. Conley PhD, Monica L.Kasting PhD
3. Very well Family -10 ways to help your teen deal with a break-up By Amy Morin.
4. Prevalence and stability of mental disorders among young adults: findings from a longitudinal study. Kristin Gustavson et al

BIBLIOGRAPHY

Oxfordreference.com
GP notebook
NHS choices
WebMD
Helpguide.org

ABOUT THE AUTHOR

Dr. Sheun Ade-Alade BSc, MBCHB, MRCGP, DRCOG is a medical doctor, a UK-based GP (general practitioner) with experience working across two continents, Africa and Europe, for the last thirteen years.

She has an interest in lifestyle medicine, women and adolescent health. She works closely with youths to help them build mental health resilience and get them to where they are meant to be. She does this through consultations, lectures and workshops.

Her passion for adolescent health inspired her to write this book.

Oluwaseun can be contacted at thebig5ofyouthwellness@gmail.com

Printed in Great Britain
by Amazon

85442107R00072